Belly fat
20 Steps on how to lose belly fat in 30 days

Olivia peters

Table of contents

You want to be Healthy, Lean, And lose that annoying fat around your bellies!

People are fighting with stubborn belly fat all over the world. You don't have to belong to them, though! Are you prepared to commit to losing weight and being sexier? Are you prepared to lose that harmful tummy fat? Are you prepared to flaunt a figure that makes you proud on the beach?
This book explains 20   tried-and-true methods for getting a flat stomach and losing belly fat quickly and naturally. In just one month, you might reduce your belly fat by up to four or five inches!.
examination of all the ways you can improve your own gut health. information that will help you get that flat belly you've always wanted!

Get ready to finally look amazing in a bikini and have a flat belly and toned tummy thanks to this book's instructions!

Download this book right away and take action today!

Step1

Dumbbell Goblet Squats

You start this exercise by vertically holding a dumbbell by the middle of your chest. Squat down until your thighs are parallel to the ground while maintaining a firm core. As you push through your heels and hips to rise back up, engage your quadriceps and glutes at the top. As you rise up one-fourth of the way. 3–4 sets of 12–15 reps should be completed.

Step 2

Band Rows

Wrap a resistance band around a solid object, such as a pole or a beam, to prepare for band rowing. Take two steps backwards after grabbing the band firmly with both hands to increase tension. Drive your elbows back, engage your shoulder blades, and maintain a tight core. Finally, extend your arms fully to complete the stretch. Finish three or four sets of 15 repetitions.

Step 3

Dumbbell Pushups

Put a set of dumbbells in front of you, then get into a pushup or high plank position. Hold the dumbbells in your hands. As you lower your body until it is only an inch or two off the ground, keep your hips up, your chest out, and your abs tight. Push yourself back up and finish by flexing your pecs and triceps. 3–4 sets of 10–15 reps should be completed.

Step 4

Bulgarian Split Squats

Beginning with a dumbbell in each hand while standing tall, perform a Bulgarian split squat. Place one foot firmly on a couch or exercise bench. With your other foot, advance a couple of feet toward the bench. Lower yourself into a split squat under control. Almost touch the ground with your rear knee. Push yourself back up while engaging your glutes and quadriceps. With each leg, perform three to four sets of ten repetitions.

Step 5

Single-Leg Dumbbell Hip Thrusts

With your legs supporting your core (which should be suspended in the air), you will position your back on a training bench for the single-leg dumbbell hip thrust. Dumbbells should be placed on top of one of your legs. As you lower your body by bending at the waist, maintain a tight core. Push through your heel to extend your hip upward as you stand back up. Prior to the following rep, controllably lower your leg after two seconds of intense top-end squeeze. With each leg, complete three to four sets of 10 to 15 repetitions.

Step 6

Plank Shoulder Taps

For this exercise, assume a pushup or high plank position while keeping your hips raised and your shoulders aligned with your wrists. As you extend one arm toward the opposing shoulder, your core should continue to be tight. After tapping that shoulder, lower your arm back down and repeat the process with the other arm. Maintain a straight spine and tight glutes. Work each arm for three to four sets of eight to ten repetition

Step 7

Cross-Body Mountain Climbers

Assume a pushup to complete the final workout, cross-body mountain climbers. Your shoulders should be in line with your wrists, and your feet should be fully extended. Flex your obliques as you drive one knee toward the opposing elbow while maintaining a tight core. Then, move the other leg through the motion while returning your first to the pushup position. Maintain tension in your core as you back and forth while doing this. With each leg, complete three to four sets of ten repetitions

Step 8

Medicine Ball Slam

Your feet should be shoulder-width apart while you hold the ball above your head.
As forcefully as you can, slam the ball on the ground. Repeat after catching the rebound.

step 9

Burpee

Place your feet shoulder-width apart as you stand. Your palms should be roughly shoulder-width apart on the floor when you squat down. Kick your legs back into a pushup stance, execute a pushup, swiftly reverse the motion, and leap once you are standing. It's one rep.

Step 10

Kettlebell Swing

Holding a kettlebell down in front of you at arms' length with both hands, squat at the hips. As you "hike" the kettlebell between your legs, lean back slightly.
Next, tighten your glutes, firmly protrude your hips forward, and swing the weight up to shoulder level. Between your legs, turn the motion around and repeat.

Step11

Treadmill Sprints

Sprint for 20 seconds and then rest for 40 seconds for the first fifteen sets, and then gradually increase the work-to-rest ratio.Increase the inclination on a treadmill, then sprint for the allocated time.

Step12

Thrusters

Hold two dumbbells or kettlebells by their handles so that the weight is on your back shoulder.

Keep your legs parallel to your shoulders as you squat down with a slight bend in your knees. Lift the kettlebells above your head by driving through your legs, straightening them, and extending your arms at the same time. Squat and do it again.

Step 13

Skaters

Standing with your legs spread by your shoulders. Jump to one side of the mat, bending one leg at a little angle behind the supporting leg.Return to your feet, then leap to the other side of your mat.

Land on the back leg of the other leg after shifting your weight.

Step 14

Tuck Jumps

Kneel down while standing with your feet hip-width apart and raise your arms overhead.

Bent more deeply and spring straight up, lifting your knees to touch your outstretched hands.

Make sure to lightly land and to keep your knees bent.

Step 15

Froggers

Put your hands on the ground between your feet while squatting.Put your legs back together and perform a press-up.

Return to the low-squat position by reversing the motion. One rep, then.

Step 16

High Knees

Place your feet hip-width apart as you stand. Your right knee should be brought up to your chest.Lifting your left knee to your chest while bending your right knee.Continue the exercise by switching legs and running or sprinting at a fast pace.

Step 17

Devil's Press

Holding two dumbbells, drop down into a press-up position and lower your chest to the ground.Press back up and quickly jump your legs back towards your chest landing with your dumbbells between your legs.As you begin to stand back up, use the momentum to swing the weights between your legs, then explosively overhead.Lower under control, back to the ground and repeat.

Step 18

Dumbell Overhead Lunge

The motion enlists your butt and back.Grab a set of dumbbells that weigh between medium and light. Your palms should face one another as you press the dumbbells overhead. Avoid craning your shoulders up toward your ears.Lunge forward, hold for a moment, then step your feet together while extending your rear leg. As you move ahead, alternate your legs.

Step 19

Squat Jumps

Place your feet hip-width apart as you stand. To push your butt back and lower yourself until your thighs are parallel to the floor, hinge at the hips.In order to leap as high as you can off the ground, press your feet firmly into the ground. When you land, let your knees bend to a 45-degree angle, then immediately squat down again and jump again

Step 20

Broad Jump

Set yourself into a squat with your feet shoulder-width apart.Bring your legs forward to provide more momentum as you bring your arms back and use them to go ahead. Jump as high as you can, then land with your knees bent.Place your hands by your sides and stand with your feet together. Jump up just enough to spread your feet wide and simultaneously raise your arms above your head.Quickly reverse the motion and then repeat without halting.